Standard Macrobiotic Diet

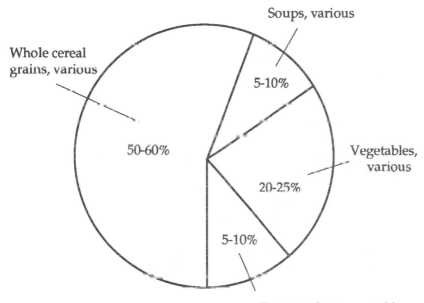

Soups, various

Whole cereal grains, various

5-10%

50-60%

Vegetables, various

20-25%

5-10%

Beans and sea vegetables, various

Plus occasional supplementary foods:
Fish and seafood, using less fatty varieties
Seasonal fruits, cooked, dried, and fresh
Nuts and seeds, various
Naturally processed seasonings, condiments, pickles, and garnishes
Naturally sweetened snacks and desserts
Natural nonaromatic and nonstimulant beverages, various

Resources

The Kushi Institute — A center for macrobiotic studies located in the Berkshire mountains of western Massachusetts with affiliates in Amsterdam and Milan and extension programs in various North American cities offers ongoing seminars and programs in macrobiotic dietary practice and way of life. The K.I.'s most popular program — the seven-day Macrobiotic Residential Seminar — provides an introduction to the standard diet for individuals and families, including daily cooking classes, classes in theory and practice, and exercise and self-reflection. For information, contact the Kushi Institute, Box 7, Becket, MA 01223 (413) 623-5741.

One Peaceful World — One Peaceful World is an international information network and friendship society of individuals, families, educational centers, organic farmers, teachers, parents and children, authors and artists, homemakers and business people, and others devoted to the realization of one healthy, peaceful world. Activities include educational and spiritual tours, assemblies and forums, international food aid and development, and publishing. For membership information and a copy of the current newsletter, contact: One Peaceful World, Box 10, Becket MA 01223 (413) 623-2322.

Michio Kushi, leader of the international macrobiotic community, lectures and gives seminars around the world on diet, health, philosophy, and culture and has guided thousands of individuals and families to greater health and happiness. Founder and president of the East West Foundation, the Kushi Foundation, and One Peaceful World and author of numerous books, he and his wife, Aveline, live in Brookline and Becket, Massachusetts.

Standard Macrobiotic Diet

By Michio Kushi

One Peaceful World Press
Becket, Massachusetts

Note to the Reader:

The guidelines in this book are for those in usual good health. It is essential that any reader who has any reason to suspect illness contact a physician promptly and seek the guidance of a medical doctor, nutritionist, or other appropriate health care professional. Neither this nor any other book should be used as a substitute for professional medical care or treatment.

Standard Macrobiotic Diet
© 1992 by Michio Kushi

Published by One Peaceful World, Becket, Massachusetts, U.S.A.

For further information on mail-order sales, wholesale or retail discounts, distribution, translations, and foreign rights, please contact the publisher:

One Peaceful World Press
P.O. Box 10
308 Leland Road
Becket, MA 01223
U.S.A.

Telephone (413) 623-2322
Fax (413) 623-8827

First Edition: January 1992
10 9 8 7 6 5 4 3 2

ISBN 0-9628528-2-1

Printed in U.S.A.

Contents

Sample Recipes   51

Appendixes   59

Introduction

The Standard Macrobiotic Diet has been practiced widely throughout history by all major civilizations and cultures in various modified styles. It is based not only on nutritional balance but also on a deep understanding of biological and spiritual evolution, present-day environmental and atmospheric conditions, the relation of the earth to the sun and other celestial bodies, ancestral tradition and heritage, affordability and other economic factors, and natural storageability and other practical considerations. In modern times, this dietary approach sometimes has been misunderstood because of a lack of information and a lack of basic understanding of ecology, human tradition and culture, and the order of nature.

Actual macrobiotic dietary practice is very broad. The guidelines presented here have been observed by millions and millions of human beings for thousands of years, contributing to health, happiness, and harmony with the earth for endless generations. In recent times, this way of eating has been exercised under the name of macrobiotics by hundreds of thousands of individuals and families wishing to attain better health and create well being within modern society.

Standard macrobiotic dietary practice is not a set, rigid diet but rather a commonsense, flexible pattern of eating that differs according to climate, environment, condition of health, sex, age, activity level, and personal need. The goal of macrobiotics is freedom — the ability to create and realize whatever we want in this life as part of our endless spiritual journey in the infinite universe. Standard macrobiotic dietary practice provides almost limitless variety and choice to prepare healthful, delicious, beautiful food suited to our unique requirements and needs.

The key principle is the use of whole cereal grains (including brown rice, barley, millet, corn, and others) as staple, central food. Day to day, meal to meal, all around the world, every previous culture and civilization has recognized the importance of whole grains as the staff of life. In modern society, grain has been largely replaced by meat, poultry, dairy food, and other animal food — with consequent harm to physical, mental, social, environmental, and spiritual health.

To reverse this trend toward biological and spiritual degeneration, modern society is beginning to rediscover the central importance of whole grains (including partial forms such as fiber and bran). In the last several years, all of the major medical and scientific associations around the world have issued dietary guidelines calling for substantial increases in whole grains, vegetables, beans, and other whole natural foods and corresponding decreases in meat, poultry, eggs, dairy food, sugar and other refined carbohydrates, and highly processed, chemicalized foods.

Macrobiotics has been on the leading edge of the current dietary revolution. However, macrobiotics is not only a healthful and orderly way of eating. It encompasses a whole lifestyle which respects diverse human traditions, ancestral spirit, natural change, and the order of the universe, with the spirit of fostering human development and creating One Peaceful World. The goal of macrobiotics is to preserve the human race and to create a new species — *homo spiritus* — which can develop endlessly toward new levels of health, happiness, and peace.

I hope that this handbook will serve as an introduction to the macrobiotic dietary approach and way of life. I am grateful to my wife, Aveline, for the recipes at the end of this book; to my associates Alex and Gale Jack and Edward and Wendy Esko of One Peaceful World Press for editing and publishing this volume; and to my grandson, Yogen, for his advice on behalf of the next generation.

Michio Kushi
Becket, Massachusetts
Autumn, 1991

Part I
Principles of
Macrobiotic Diet

Nutritional Characteristics

In comparison with currently practiced dietary habits in modern society, Standard Macrobiotic Dietary Practice has the following nutritional characteristics:

1. More complex carbohydrates, less simple sugars.

2. More vegetable-quality protein, less animal food protein.

3. Less overall consumption of fat — more unsaturated fat and less saturated fat.

4. More consideration in balancing various vitamins, minerals, and other nutritional factors.

5. Use of more organically grown, natural quality food utilizing more traditional food processing techniques and less artificially and chemically processed foods.

6. Consumption of more food in whole form as much as possible, and less refined and partial foods.

7. Consumption of more food rich in natural fiber and less food which has been devitalized.

Scientific and Medical Guidelines

Standard Macrobiotic Dietary Practice shares a similar orientation to the dietary guidelines issued by the following national and international scientific and medical associations:

1. The United States Congress, Senate Select Committee on Nutrition and Human Needs: *Dietary Goals for the United States* (1977).

2. The U.S. Surgeon-General's report: *Healthy People: Health Promotion and Disease Prevention* (1979).

3. A 472-page report by the National Academy of Sciences: *Diet, Nutrition, and Cancer* (1982).

4. Dietary guidelines of the American Heart Association (1985), the American Cancer Society (1984), the American Medical Association (1987), the Canadian Department of National Health and Welfare (1977), the National Advisory Committee on Nutritional Education of the United Kingdom (1983), the Panel on Nutrition and Prevention of Diseases in Japan (1983), the Japanese Ministry of Health and Welfare (1985), and other scientific and medical bodies.

5. A 749-page report by the National Academy of Sciences: *Diet and Health: The Implications for Reducing Chronic Disease* (1989).

6. Guidelines issued by the U.S. Department of Agriculture and the Department of Health and Human Services: *Dietary Guidelines for Americans* (1990).

7. An international study sponsored by the U.S. National Cancer Institute and the Chinese Institute of Nutrition and Food Hygiene: *Diet, LifeStyle, and Mortality in China* (1990).

8. The guidelines of the Physicians Committee for Responsible Medicine (1991).

9. The Eating Right Pyramid under consideration by the U.S. Department of Agriculture (1991).

10. Guidelines by the World Health Organization (1982, 1990).

Standard Macrobiotic Dietary Practice

The Standard Macrobiotic Diet is not designed for any particular person, nor for a particular condition. It is designed for the general purpose of maintaining physical and psychological health and the well-being of society in general. It further serves, in many instances, to prevent degenerative diseases and promote possible recovery from disorders.

These dietary guidelines have been practiced daily for more than twenty years by hundreds of thousands of macrobiotic individuals and families throughout the world. Furthermore, the same or similar dietary practice has been observed traditionally in many cultures and civilizations throughout the world for thousands and thousands of years.

The following guidelines are designed primarily for people living in a temperate climate zone and cover the majority of the world's people. Countries and regions that experience the regular change of four seasons include most of North America, Europe (including most of the Soviet Union), China, Japan, and temperate parts of Africa, Latin America, and Australia.

The Standard Diet differs, and modification is required, for people living in a tropical and semitropical climate as well as a polar and semipolar climatic region. This includes equatorial regions of the world in Latin America, Africa, South Asia and Southeast Asia, the Middle East, Oceania, and other warm regions and the Arctic, Siberia, Mongolia, and other cold regions.

The Appendix summarizes suggested dietary modifications for these regions.

Principles of Dietary Practice

The Standard Macrobiotic Diet:

1. Considers biological evolutionary processes, particularly human needs.

2. Respects centuries-old traditionally and universally practiced dietary customs of different cultures and civilizations throughout the world.

3. Adapts to the climatic, seasonal, and environmental differences prevailing.

4. Considers social and economical requirements which can be practiced widely throughout the world at a reasonable cost.

5. Satisfies the nutritional balance and requirements for human needs.

6. Benefits physical and psychological health, preventing disorders in some instances and, if possible, promoting recovery.

7. Requires modification and adjustment for personal and individual needs by securing varieties in the kinds of foods selected and the method of preparation and cooking.

8. Secures family health and harmony as well as a peaceful mind with energetic physical conditions for the well-being of society.

9. Is based upon the use of organically-grown natural products as much as possible with minimization of heavily chemicalized and artificially processed foods.

Variety of Foods

The practice of the Standard Macrobiotic Diet consists of a wide variety of foods:

Whole Grains and Grain Products

Soup

Vegetables

Beans and Bean Products

Sea Vegetables

Fish and Seafood

Fruit

Pickles

Nuts and Seeds

Snacks

Condiments

Garnishes

Seasonings

Desserts

Beverages

These foods have been traditionally used and commonly consumed throughout the world. The food selection, variety of food preparation, spectrum of cooking techniques, and wide range of combinations of foods serve to secure varying human requirements which differ according to the season, activity level, sex, and age, as well as environment, climate, tradition, and custom.

Variety of Cooking and Preparation Methods

For variety, aspects of daily cooking may be changed in the following ways:

1. The selection of foods within each category: whole grains, soups, vegetables, beans, sea vegetables, condiments, pickles, and beverages.

2. The methods of cooking: boiling, steaming, sautéing, frying, pressure cooking, and others.

3. The ways of cutting vegetables: large chunks, medium slices, slivers, quarters, halves, half-moons, chrysanthemums, irregular shapes, etc., in addition to grating and mashing.

4. The amount of water used.

5. The amount of seasoning and condiments used.

6. The kind of seasoning and condiments used.

7. The length of cooking time (do not overcook or pressure-cook vegetables, however).

8. The use of higher or lower flame in cooking.

9. The combination of foods and dishes.

10. Seasonal cooking adjustments.

Food Preparation

Macrobiotic cooking is unique. The ingredients are simple though varied and cooking is the key to producing meals that are nutritious, tasty, and attractive. The cook has the ability to change the quality of the food. More cooking, the use of pressure, salt, heat, and time makes the energy of food more concentrated, while quick cooking and less salt preserve the lighter quality of the food. A good cook controls the health of those for whom she or he cooks by varying the cooking style often. Methods of cooking and food preparation include:

Regular Use

Pressure cooking
Boiling
Steaming
Waterless cooking
Soup
Pickling
Oil sautéing
Water sautéing
Pressing

Occasional Use

Stir-frying
Raw
Deep-frying
Tempura
Broiling
Baking
Roasting
Drying

Part II

Summary of Daily Dietary Recommendations

1. Whole Cereal Grains

On the average, 50 percent by volume of every meal is recommended to include cooked, organically grown, whole cereal grains prepared in a variety of ways. Whole cereal grains include brown rice, barley, millet, oats, corn, rye, wheat, buckwheat, and other grains. Please note that a portion of this amount may consist of noodles or pasta, unyeasted whole grain breads, and other partially processed whole cereal grains. However, whole grain prepared in whole form should form the center of every meal.

2. Soups

About 5 to 10 percent of our daily food intake may include soup made with vegetables, sea vegetables (wakame or kombu), grains or beans. Seasonings are usually miso or soy sauce (shoyu). The flavor should not be too salty and be suitable to personal conditions and taste.

3. Vegetables

About 20 to 30 percent of our daily intake may include organic vegetables (locally grown if available). Preferably, the majority are

15

cooked in various styles (e.g., sautéed with a small amount of sesame or corn oil, steamed, boiled, and sometimes prepared using soy sauce or light sea salt as a seasoning). A smaller portion may be eaten as raw salad. Pickled vegetables without highly stimulant spice may also be used daily in small volume.

It is advisable that green leafy, round, and root vegetables be taken daily. Vegetables for daily use include, as examples: *green leafy vegetables*: bok choy, Chinese cabbage, collard greens, kale, leeks, mustard greens, parsley, scallions, turnip greens, and watercress. *Round vegetables*: acorn squash, broccoli, Brussel sprouts, butternut squash, buttercup squash, cabbage, cauliflower, onion, pumpkin, rutabaga, and turnip. *Root vegetables*: burdock, carrots, daikon, lotus root, parsnips, and radish.

4. Beans and Sea Vegetables

About 5 to 10 percent of our daily diet includes cooked beans and sea vegetables. The most suitable beans for regular use are azuki beans, chickpeas, and lentils. Other beans may be used on occasion. Bean products such as tofu, tempeh, and natto may also be used often. Sea vegetables such as nori, wakame, kombu, hiziki, arame, dulse, sea palm, agar-agar, Irish moss, and other edible sea vegetables may be prepared in a variety of ways. They can be cooked with beans or vegetables, used in soups, or served separately as side dishes, flavored with a moderate amount of soy sauce (shoyu), sea salt, brown rice vinegar, umeboshi plum, umeboshi vinegar, and others.

5. Occasional Foods

If needed or desired, 1 to 3 times a week, about 5 to 15 percent of that day's food consumption can include fresh nonfat white-meat fish such as flounder, sole, cod, carp, halibut, trout, and others.

Fruit or fruit desserts, including fresh, dried, and cooked fruits, may also be served two or three times a week. Local and organically grown fruits are preferred. If you live in a temperate climate, avoid tropical and semitropical fruit and eat, instead, temperate climate fruits such as apples, pears, plums, peaches, apricots, cherries, berries, and melons. Frequent use of fruit juice is not advisable. However, occasional consumption in warmer weather may be appropri-

16

ate, depending on your health.

Lightly roasted nuts and seeds such as pumpkin, sesame, and sunflower seeds, peanuts, walnuts, and pecans may be enjoyed as a snack.

Rice syrup, barley malt, and amasake may be used as a sweetener; brown rice vinegar or umeboshi vinegar may be used occasionally for a sour taste.

6. Beverages

Recommended daily beverages include roasted bancha twig tea, bancha stem tea, roasted brown rice tea, roasted barley tea, dandelion tea, and cereal grain coffee. Any traditional tea that does not have an aromatic fragrance or a stimulating effect can be used. You may also drink a moderate amount of water (preferably spring or well water of good quality) but not iced.

7. Food to Avoid for Better Health

The following are preferably avoided in a temperate, four-season climate:

Meat, animal fat, eggs, poultry, dairy products (including butter yogurt, ice cream, milk, and cheese), refined sugars, chocolate, molasses, honey, other simple sugars and foods treated with them, and vanilla.

Tropical or semitropical fruits and fruit juices, soda, artificial drinks and beverages, coffee, colored tea, black tea, green tea, and all aromatic stimulating teas such as mint or peppermint tea.

Potatoes (including sweet potatoes and yams), tomatoes, eggplant, peppers, asparagus, spinach, avocado, and other vegetables of tropical or semitropical origin. Mayonnaise and other oily dressings are better avoided, as well as palm oil, coconut oil, and other tropical oils.

All artificially colored, preserved, sprayed, or chemically treated foods. All refined and polished grains, flours, and their derivatives. Mass-produced industrialized food including all canned, frozen, and irradiated foods.

Hot spices and herbs, any aromatic stimulating food or food accessory, artificial vinegar and artificial soy sauce, and strong alcoholic beverages.

8. Additional Suggestions

Cooking oil should be vegetable quality only. To maintain usual good health, it is preferable to use unrefined sesame (dark or light) oil or stoneground unrefined corn oil in moderate amounts.

Salt should be naturally processed, white sea salt. Traditionally, non-chemicalized soy sauce (shoyu) and miso (especially two-to-three year naturally fermented barley miso) may also be used as seasonings.

Recommended condiments include: gomashio (12 to 18 parts roasted sesame seeds to 1 part roasted sea salt, both crushed and well mixed), sea vegetable powder, umeboshi plums, tekka root vegetable condiment, soy sauce (moderate use, use only in cooking for mild flavoring, and avoid wheat-free or low-sodium soy sauce), pickles (made using bran, miso, soy sauce, or salt), sauerkraut.

You may have meals regularly, two to three times per day, as much as you want, provided the proportion is generally correct and chewing is thorough. No regular eating at night is recommended. Avoid eating for approximately three hours before sleeping.

9. The Importance of Cooking

Proper cooking is very important for health. Everyone should learn to cook either by attending classes or under the guidance of an experienced macrobiotic cook.

10. Special Advice

The guidelines presented in this book are general suggestions. These suggestions may require modification depending on your special condition and personal needs. Of course, any serious condition should be closely monitored by the appropriate medical, nutritional, and health professional.

Along with beginning to change your diet, we invite you to attend any of our regular study programs or seminars and to meet personally with a qualified macrobiotic teacher as well as attend cooking classes. Please see the Resource Section at the front for recommended classes and further studies.

Part III

Standard Macrobiotic Dietary Practice

Whole Grains

Within the Standard Macrobiotic Diet, especially in a temperate climate, whole grains are an essential part of the daily diet. They comprise between 40 and 60 percent (average 50 percent) of the daily food intake by volume.

Use of Whole Grains and Grain Products

Regular Use

Short-grain brown rice
Medium-grain brown rice
Long-grain brown rice
  (in subtropical regions)
Whole barley
Pearl barley (hato mugi)

Corn
Whole wheat
Millet
Buckwheat
Whole oats
Rye
Other whole grains traditionally
  eaten in a four-season climate

Occasional Use

Sweet brown rice
Wild rice
Mochi (pounded sweet rice)
Cracked wheat (bulghur)
Steel-cut oats
Rolled oats
Corn grits
Rye flakes
Couscous
Quinoa
Amaranth
Teff
Other grains and grain products

Occasional Use Flour Products

Whole wheat noodles and pasta
Udon noodles (whole wheat)
Somen noodles (whole wheat)
Soba noodles (buckwheat)
Unyeasted whole wheat bread or whole rye bread
Chapatis, tortillas, pancakes, and other flat breads
Fu (puffed wheat gluten
Seitan (wheat gluten)
Cornmeal
Other flour products

Kinds of Whole Grains and Grain Products

Brown Rice

Brown rice — short, medium, and long grain
Genuine brown rice cream (homemade rather than store-bought)
Puffed brown rice
Brown rice noodles
Brown rice bread
Brown rice crackers
Brown rice flour products
Brown rice flakes

Sweet Brown Rice

Sweet brown rice grain
Mochi (pounded sweet brown rice)
Sweet brown rice flour products
Sweet rice crackers and cookies

Wild Rice

Wild rice grain

Whole Wheat

Whole wheat berries
Whole wheat bread
Whole wheat chapatis and tortillas (flat bread)
Whole wheat noodles and pasta
Whole wheat flakes
Whole wheat flour products, such as crackers, matzos, muffins,
    bagels, biscuits, and others
Couscous
Bulghur
Cracked wheat
Seitan (wheat gluten)
Fu (baked puffed wheat gluten)

Barley

Barley grain
Pearled barley (partially polished barley)
Pearl barley (hato mugi)
Puffed barley
Barley bread
Barley flour products

Rye

Rye grain
Rye bread
Rye flakes
Rye flour products

Millet

Millet grain
Millet flour products
Puffed millet

Oats

Whole oats
Steel-cut oats (Scotch oats)
Rolled oats
Oatmeal
Oat flakes
Oat flour products
Puffed oats

Corn

Corn on the cob
Corn grits
Cornmeal
Tortillas
Arepas (corn balls)
Corn flour products such as cornbread, muffins, dumplings
Puffed corn
Popcorn
Corn nuts

Buckwheat

Buckwheat groats
Kasha
Buckwheat noodles and pasta (soba and others)
Buckwheat flour products such as pancakes

Other Traditional Grains and Grain Products

Cooking Styles for Whole Grains

Pressure cooking
Boiling
Steaming
Baking
Frying such as fried rice, fried noodles
Roasting
Other traditionally practiced and commonly used cooking styles

Cooking Varieties for Whole Grains

Cook with a pinch of sea salt
Occasionally cook with vegetables
Occasionally cook with beans
Occasionally cook with other grains
Occasionally cook with sea vegetables
Occasionally cook with fish or seafood (paella)
Occasionally cook in soup with vegetables and sea vegetables
Cook as a soft breakfast porridge
Occasionally cook as croquettes or dumplings
Occasionally cook as noodles or pasta or as bread and baked goods
Other traditionally practiced and commonly used cooking varieties

Seasonings That Can Be Used
When Cooking Whole Grains

Season with a pinch of sea salt
Season with a touch of soy sauce (shoyu)
Season with miso (fermented soybean and grain paste)
Season with kombu or other sea vegetable
Season with pickled umeboshi plum
Season with gravy or a sauce
Other traditionally practiced and commonly used seasonings

Soup

The Standard Macrobiotic Diet recommends, under normal circumstances, a daily average consumption of one or two cups or bowls of soup every day.

Kinds of Soup

Miso soup with vegetables, sea vegetables, grains, etc.
Clear soup made with soy sauce (shoyu)
Light broth for noodles or pasta
Vegetable soup
Vegetable and sea vegetable (usually wakame or kombu) soup
Bean and vegetable soup
Grain and vegetable soup
Fish and vegetable soup
Fish and vegetable and sea vegetable soup
Bread and vegetable soup
Dumpling and vegetable soup
Soup stewed with grains, vegetables, beans, sea vegetables and/or fish and seafood
Other traditionally used and commonly consumed soups

Kinds of Vegetables Usually used in Soup

Acorn squash	Jinenjo
Bok Choy	Kale
Broccoli	Leeks
Brussel sprouts	Lambsquarters
Burdock	Lotus root
Buttercup squash	Mustard greens
Butternut squash	Mushrooms
Cabbage	Onion
Carrots	Parsley
Carrot tops	Patty pan squash
Celery	Parsnip

Celery root
Cauliflower
Chives
Chinese cabbage
Coltsfoot
Daikon
Daikon greens
Dandelion leaves
Dandelion roots
Endive
Escarole
Green beans
Hokkaido pumpkin
Hubbard squash

Radish
Red Cabbage
Rutabaga
Scallions
Shiitake mushrooms
Snap beans
Snow peas
Sprouts
Summer squash
Turnips
Turnip greens
Watercress
Wax beans
Other vegetables traditionally
    used and consumed

Kinds of Grains Used in Soup

Brown rice
Corn
Millet
Barley
Oats
Buckwheat
Wholewheat noodles and pasta
Wholewheat dumplings
Buckwheat noodles and pasta
Couscous
Mochi (pounded sweet rice)
Other traditionally used and consumed grains

Kinds of Beans Usually Used in Soup

Aduki beans
Black beans
Chickpeas (garbanzo beans)
Lentils
Split peas
Other beans

Kinds of Sea Vegetables
Most Popularly Used in Soup

Wakame sea vegetable
Nori sea vegetable
Kombu sea vegetable
Dulse sea vegetable
Other edible sea vegetables

Fish and Seafood Occasionally Used in Soup

Carp
Cod
Dried fish
Small dried fish (iriko)
Flounder
Haddock
Herring
Scrod
Snapper
Sole
Trout
Other white-meat fish

Occasional Use Seafood:

Cherrystone clam
Littleneck clam
Other clams
Crab
Lobster
Octopus
Oysters
Shrimp

Seasonings for Soup

Miso (fermented soybean and grain paste)
Soy sauce (shoyu)
Sea salt
Sesame or corn oil (occasionally)
Other traditionally used and commonly consumed condiments

Garnishes for Soup

Grated ginger root (occasional use)
Nori sea vegetable

Parsley
Scallions
Onions
Others

Vegetables

A variety of vegetable dishes prepared in a variety of cooking styles comprises about 25 to 30 percent of the daily food intake.

Kinds of Vegetables

Regular Use

Green Leafy

Bok choy
Carrot tops
Chinese cabbage
Chives
Collard greens
Dandelion leaves
Kale
Leeks
Mustard greens
Parsley
Scallions
Turnip greens
Watercress
Others

Root

Burdock
Carrots
Daikon
Jinenjo

Round

Acorn squash
Broccoli
Brussel sprouts
Butternut squash
Buttercup squash
Cabbage
Cauliflower
Hubbard squash
Hokkaido pumpkin
Onion
Pumpkin
Red cabbage
Rutabaga
Turnip
Others

Lotus root
Parsnips
Radish
Others

Fungi
Shiitake mushrooms

Occasional Use Vegetables

Beets	Lambsquarters
Celery	Mushrooms
Chives	Patty pan squash
Coltsfoot	Romaine lettuce
Cucumber	Salsify
Endive	Snap beans
Escarole	Snow peas
Garlic	Sprouts
Green beans	Summer squash
Green peas	Wax beans
Iceberg lettuce	Winter melon
Jerusalem artichoke	Zucchini
Kohlrabi	

Wild grasses that have been used widely for centuries
Other traditionally used and commonly consumed vegetables

Cooking Styles for Vegetables

Raw salad

Pressed salad (salt and pressure added for a few hours to a few days)

Boiled salad (adding vegetables to boiling water and cooking for 1 to 3 minutes)

Boiling

Baking

Broiling

Steaming

Water sautéing

Oil sautéing (using a small volume of vegetable quality oil)

Waterless cooking (cooking with a small volume of water and high steam until the water evaporates

Deep-frying (usually with a batter made of unrefined wholewheat flour)

Pickling

Other traditionally used and commonly practiced cooking styles

Seasoning for Vegetable Dishes

Miso (fermented soybean and grain paste)
Soy sauce (shoyu)
Sea salt
Mirin (fermented sweetener made of sweet brown rice)
Brown rice vinegar
Umeboshi plum (pickled plum) vinegar
Oil (sesame, corn, mustard seed, safflower, sunflower, olive, and
other traditionally consumed oils)

Styles of Preparing Vegetables

Cooked separately
Cooked together and served as a casserole
Cooked in soup
Cooked with grains
Cooked with beans or bean products
Cooked with sea vegetables
Used as an ingredient in sushi
Served with noodle or pasta dishes
Cooked and served with fish or seafood
Used as an ingredient in dessert dishes

Beans

The Standard Macrobiotic Diet recommends a moderate volume of beans or bean products be taken daily, about 5 to 10 percent of daily food intake by volume.

Kinds and Use of Beans and Bean Products

Regular Use

Azuki beans

Chickpeas (garbanzo beans)
Lentils (green or brown)
Black soybeans

Tofu (fresh soybean curd)
Dried tofu
Natto (fermented soybeans)
Okara (residue in making tofu)
Tempeh (fermented soybeans)

Occasional Use

Black-eyed peas
Black soybeans
Black turtle beans
Great northern beans
Kidney beans
Lentils (red)
Lima beans
Mung beans
Navy beans
Pinto beans
Soybeans
Split peas and whole dried peas
Other traditionally used and commonly consumed beans

Cooking Styles for Beans

Boiling
Pressure cooking
Roasting
Fermenting
Steaming
Other traditionally used and commonly practiced cooking styles

Cooking Varieties for Beans

Cook beans with a small amount of sea salt or miso (usually added
     toward the end of cooking)
Cook beans with sea vegetables, usually kombu (10%)

Cook beans with carrots or onions (20%)
Cook beans with acorn or buttercup squash (30-50%)
Cook beans with chestnuts (10-30%)
Cook beans with vegetables
Cook beans with grains (10%)
Cook beans as a dessert sweetened with barley or rice malt
Other traditionally used and commonly practiced cooking varieties

Seasonings Generally Used for Beans

Sea salt
Miso (fermented soybean and grain paste)
Soy sauce (shoyu)
Tamari
Barley malt or rice malt
Oil (vegetable quality)

Garnishes Generally Used with Beans

Grated ginger root
Grated fresh daikon
Grated fresh radish
Grated fresh horseradish
Chopped fresh scallions
Chopped fresh onions
Brown rice vinegar
Sweet brown rice vinegar
Mustard
Umeboshi vinegar
Other traditionally used and commonly consumed garnishes

Sea Vegetables

The Standard Macrobiotic Diet recommends sea vegetables to be consumed daily as a small side dish, in soups, vegetables dishes, or in bean or grain dishes. Amount consumed averages about 3 to 5 percent of daily food intake by volume.

Kinds of Sea Vegetables

Kombu
Wakame
Nori
Arame
Hiziki
Dulse
Sea Palm
Agar-Agar
Irish moss
Mekabu
Nekabu
Other edible sea vegetables that have been traditionally used and
   commonly consumed

Cooking Styles for Sea Vegetables

Boiling
Steaming
Sautéing
Deep-frying
Toasting or roasting
Pickling
In waterless cooking
Drying
Raw

Cooking Varieties for Sea Vegetables

Cook sea vegetables alone
Cook sea vegetables with beans
Cook sea vegetables with grains
Cook sea vegetables in vegetable dishes
Cook sea vegetables as gelatin
Cook sea vegetables in sauces
Cook sea vegetables with fish or seafood

Fish and Seafood

The Standard Macrobiotic Diet recommends fish and seafood as an occasional supplement to grains, soups, vegetables, beans, sea vegetables, and beverages. The amount of fish or seafood varies according to health and personal needs and can range from once in a while to several times a week. The average, however, is two or three times a week, with the amount not exceeding 20 percent of the total volume of food consumed that day. The kinds of fish and seafood recommended are those with less saturated fat and cholesterol and those most easily digested.

Kinds of Fish and Seafood

Carp
Cod
Flounder
Haddock
Halibut
Herring
Scrod
Smelt
Snapper
Sole
Trout
Other white-meat fish
Dried fish
Small dried fish (iriko)

Occasional Use Seafood

Cherrystone clams
Littleneck clams

Other clams
Crab
Lobster
Octopus
Oysters
Shrimp

Infrequent Use Fish

Bluefish
Salmon
Sardines
Swordfish
Tuna
Other blue-skinned and red-meat varieties

Varieties of Cooking Styles for Fish and Seafood

Raw and fresh (sashimi and sushi)
Marinated
Steamed
Boiled
Baked
Broiled
Sautéed
Pan-fried
Deep-fried (tempura)
Dried and then boiled
Dried and then steamed
Dried and then baked
Fish flakes
Pickles
Smoked
Other traditionally used and commonly practiced cooking styles

Cooking Varieties for Fish and Seafood

Cooked in soup
Cooked as a separate dish
Cooked in stew
Cooked with grains (paella)
Cooked with vegetables
Cooked with sea vegetables
Used as flavoring and seasoning in soup, vegetable dishes, and other dishes
Served with raw fresh salad
Served as fish cake
Other traditionally used and commonly prepared varieties

Garnishes Used to Balance Fish and Seafood Dishes

Chopped scallions
Grated daikon
Grated radish
Grated ginger root
Green mustard paste
Grated horseradish
Shredded daikon
Raw fresh salad
Lemon
Orange
Fresh beefsteak plant leaves
Other traditionally used and commonly consumed garnishes

Seasonings for Fish and Seafood

Sea salt
Soy sauce (shoyu)
Miso (fermented soybean and grain paste)
Tamari (as seasoning or as a dipping sauce)
Ginger
Lemon
Black peppercorns
Red pepper
Rice vinegar
Umeboshi vinegar
Sesame oil, corn oil, safflower oil, mustard seed oil, olive oil
Mirin (fermented sweet rice sweetener)
Tofu sauce seasoned with some of the above ingredients
Kuzu sauce seasoned with some of the above ingredients
Oil sauce seasoned with some of the above ingredients
Other traditionally used and commonly consumed seasonings

Fruit

The Standard Macrobiotic Diet consists of the occasional consumption of fruit depending upon the climate, season, personal needs, and circumstances. All traditionally used and commonly consumed fruits growing in a temperate climate are included. The regular use of tropical fruits in a temperate climate is discouraged.

Kinds of Fruit

Apples
Apricots
Blackberries
Cantaloupe
Grapes
Grapefruit
Honeydew melon
Lemons
Mulberries
Oranges

Persimmon
Peaches
Plums
Raisins
Raspberries
Strawberries
Tangerines
Watermelon
Wild berries

Other fruit traditionally grown in a temperate climate

Variety of Serving Styles for Fruit

Fresh and raw
Fresh, raw, and soaked in lightly salted water
Grated
Boiled
Baked
Steamed
Juice as a beverage or flavoring
Preserved
Spread on bread or other baked flour products
As an ingredient in stuffing
As a dessert
As an ingredient and flavoring in kuzu or agar-agar gelatin
Baked in bread
Dried fruit as a snack, garnish, or dessert
Pickled fruit
Deep-fried fruit (in a batter)
Served as a garnish
Fermented beverages
Other traditionally used and commonly consumed serving styles

Pickles

The Standard Macrobiotic Diet recommends frequent use of pickles as a supplement to various main dishes and for the purpose of stimulating appetite and encouraging digestion. Some pickles are available in natural food stores, while many of them can be prepared at home. Some pickles are ready in a few hours, others require more pickling time — from a few days to a few seasons. Dill pickles, herb pickles, garlic pickles, spiced pickles, and vinegar pickles made with commercial apple cider vinegar or wine vinegar are preferably avoided.

Kinds of Food Often Used in Making Pickles

Burdock root
Broccoli
Cabbage
Carrots
Cauliflower
Chinese cabbage
Cucumbers
Daikon
Leeks
Lotus root
Mustard greens
Olives
Onions
Pumpkin
Radishes, red and white
Red cabbage
Scallions

Squash
Tofu
Turnips
Apricots
Anchovies
Caviar
Herring
Salmon
Sardines

Other traditionally used and commonly selected foods for making
    pickles

Methods Used in Pickling

Salt pickles
Salt and water pickles
Bran pickles
Brine pickles
Miso pickles (fermented soybean and grain sauce)
Soy sauce (shoyu) pickles
Sauerkraut
Takuan pickles
Umeboshi pickles
Other traditionally used and commonly practiced pickling methods

Nuts

The Standard Macrobiotic Diet includes occasional consumption of various kinds of nuts in the form of snacks, garnishes, or as an ingredient in desserts.

Kinds of Nuts

Almonds
Chestnuts
Filberts
Peanuts
Pecans
Pinenuts

Spanish nuts
Walnuts

Less Frequent Use

Brazil nuts
Cashews
Hazels
Macadamia nuts
Pistachio nuts
Other traditionally used and commonly consumed nuts

Variety of Serving Styles for Nuts

Roasted with sea salt
Roasted without sea salt
Roasted and sweetened with barley malt
Roasted and sweetened with rice malt
Roasted and seasoned with soy sauce (shoyu)
Ground into nut butter
Shaved and served as a topping, garnish, or ingredient in other dishes
Cooked in grain flour products such as cookies, cakes, muffins, pastries, pies, and other desserts and breads
Served with dried fruits as a snack
Other traditionally used and commonly practiced serving methods

Seeds

The Standard Macrobiotic Diet includes the occasional consumption of various seeds in various methods of preparation.

Kinds of Seeds

Black sesame seeds
White sesame seeds
Pumpkin seeds
Squash seeds
Sunflower seeds
Poppy seeds
Plum seeds
Umeboshi plum seeds
Alfalfa seeds
Other traditionally used and commonly consumed seeds

Variety of Serving Styles for Seeds

As Condiments

Dried and ground
Roasted and ground
Roasted and ground with sea salt
With umeboshi powder and sea salt
With miso (fermented soybean and grain paste)

As Snacks

Dried and served alone
Roasted and served alone
With barley malt or rice syrup
As a coating for rice balls
Baked with flour products such as cookies, crackers, breads, cakes,
    and other baked flour products
As an ingredient in candies
Other traditionally used and commonly consumed snacks

As Garnishes

Sprinkled on various dishes such as grains, soups, vegetable dishes,
    beans, fish and seafood, fruit, and desserts

Seasonings Commonly Used with Seeds

Sea salt
Soy sauce (shoyu)
Miso (fermented soybean and grain paste)
Barley malt
Rice malt
Other traditionally used and commonly consumed seasonings

Snacks

The Standard Macrobiotic Diet includes daily or occasional use
of snacks of various kinds to be consumed in reasonable and moderate amount.

Kinds of Snacks

Grain-Based Snacks

Cookies, crackers, wafers, pancakes, muffins, bread, puffed brown
  rice, barley, oats, millet, corn, popcorn
Mochi (pounded sweet rice)
Noodles and pasta
Rice balls
Rice cakes
Homemade sushi
Roasted grains
Other traditionally used and commonly consumed natural snacks

Bean-Based Snacks

Roasted beans
Boiled beans

Nut-Based Snacks

Nuts roasted and seasoned with sea salt
Nuts roasted and seasoned with soy sauce (shoyu)
Nuts roasted and seasoned with barley malt
Nuts roasted and seasoned with rice malt
Nuts used in cookies, crackers, and as an ingredient in other baked
  flour products

Seed-Based Snacks

Seeds roasted and seasoned with sea salt
Seeds roasted and seasoned with soy sauce (shoyu)
Seeds roasted and seasoned with barley malt
Seeds roasted and seasoned with rice malt
Seeds used in cookies, crackers, and as an ingredient in other baked
  flour products

Sea Vegetable-Based Snacks

Sea vegetable crackers
Baked sea vegetables

Fried sea vegetables
Sea vegetables also as an ingredient in crackers, cookies, and
other grain flour products

Fruit-Based Snacks

Fresh fruits
Cooked fruits
Dried fruits
Fruit used as an ingredient in cookies, muffins, and other grain
flour products
Other traditionally used and commonly consumed fruit snacks

Condiments

The Standard Macrobiotic Diet uses a wide variety of condiments for daily, regular, or occasional use. They are sprinkled on or added in small amount to food as an adjustment to taste, seasoning, and flavoring as well as contributing to the nutritional value of food and helping to stimulate appetite and digestion. Condiments are commonly used for grains, soups, vegetable dishes, bean dishes, and sometimes with desserts.

Kinds of Condiments

Gomashio (roasted sesame seeds and sea salt)
Sea vegetable powder
Sea vegetable powder with roasted sesame seeds
Tekka (condiment made from soybean miso, sesame oil, burdock,
lotus root, carrots, and ginger root)
Umeboshi plum (pickled plum)
Umeboshi plum and raw scallions or onions
Shio kombu (kombu cooked with soy sauce and water)
Chopped shiso leaves (pickled beefsteak plant leaves)
Roasted shiso leaves
Green nori
Dried pieces of wakame

Yellow mustard (used mainly for fish and seafood)
Green mustard (used mainly for fish and seafood)
Cooked miso with scallions or onions
Cooked nori condiment
Roasted sesame seeds
Other traditionally used and commonly consumed condiments

Seasonings

The Standard Macrobiotic Diet uses regularly, as well as occasionally, a variety of seasonings in cooking and before serving. The seasonings are all vegetable-quality, naturally processed. These seasonings have been used traditionally throughout the world. The use of seasonings should be moderate and adequate for personal needs. Commercial seasonings, spices, herbs, and other sugary, hot, pungent, aromatic seasonings are avoided. The following seasonings are commonly used within the Standard Macrobiotic Diet.

Kinds of Seasonings

Unrefined sea salt
Soy sauce (shoyu)
Miso (fermented soybean and grain paste)
    Barley miso
    Rice miso
    Soybean miso (hatcho miso)
    Sesame miso
    Other traditionally used and commonly consumed miso
Rice vinegar
Brown rice vinegar
Umeboshi vinegar
Sauerkraut brine
Mirin (fermented sweet brown rice sweetener)
Tamari
Amasake (fermented sweet brown rice beverage)
Barley malt
Rice malt

Grated ginger root
Grated daikon
Grated radish
Horseradish
Umeboshi paste
Umeboshi plum
Lemon juice
Tangerine juice
Orange juice
Freshly ground black pepper
Red pepper
Green mustard paste
Yellow mustard paste
Sesame oil
Corn oil
Safflower oil
Mustard seed oil
Olive oil
Sake (fermented rice wine)
Sake lees (residue in making sake)
Other natural seasonings that have been traditionally used

Garnishes

The Standard Macrobiotic Diet emphasizes balance of qualities, tastes, nutritional factors, and energetic harmony. For that purpose, garnishes are used in small volume frequently to balance some dishes, especially for the purpose of creating easier digestion.

Kinds of Garnishes

Grated daikon (used mainly as a garnish for fish and seafood, mochi, buckwheat noodles and pasta, natto, and tempeh)
Grated radish (used mainly the same as grated daikon)
Grated horseradish (used mainly the same as grated daikon or grated radish)
Chopped scallions (used mainly for noodle and pasta dishes, fish and seafood, natto, and tempeh)

Grated ginger, green mustard paste, freshly ground pepper, lemon pieces (used individually, mainly as a garnish for soup, noodle and pasta dishes, fish and seafood)

Red pepper, freshly ground pepper, green mustard paste (used individually, mainly for soup, noodle and pasta dishes, fish and seafood, natto, and tempeh).

Desserts

The Standard Macrobiotic Diet includes use of a variety of desserts usually served at the end of a major meal. Whenever possible, a sweet taste can be achieved with naturally sweet vegetables such as cabbage, carrots, daikon, onions, squash, pumpkins, and parsnips. Grain-based sweeteners that enter the bloodstream gradually are recommended instead of sugar, honey, molasses, or other strong simple sugars. These include barley malt, brown rice malt or syrup, and amasake. On the average, desserts are eaten two to three times a week.

Kinds of Desserts

Aduki beans sweetened with barley malt or rice malt

Aduki beans cooked with chestnuts

Aduki beans cooked with squash

Kuzu sweetened with barley malt, rice malt, fresh fruit, or dried fruit

Agar-agar cooked with barley malt, rice malt, fresh fruit, or dried fruit

Fresh fruit

Cooked fruit

Dried fruit

Dried fruit with seeds and nuts

Fruit pies including apple, peach, strawberry, berry, and other temperate climate fruits

Vegetables pies including squash, pumpkin, parsnip, and others made with naturally sweet vegetables

Fruit crunch including apple, peach, strawberry, berry, and other temperate climate fruits

Grain desserts sweetened with dried fruits, barley malt, rice malt, amasake, fresh fruit, e.g., couscous cake, Indian pudding, rice pudding, amasake pudding, and other naturally sweetened desserts

Baked flour desserts such as cookies, cakes, pies, muffins, breads, and other prepared with natural sweeteners including fruits and grain sweeteners

Beverages

The Standard Macrobiotic Diet recommends various beverages for daily, regular, or occasional consumption. The amount of beverage intake varies according to the individual's needs and the climate change. Beverage consumption should comfortably satisfy the person's desire for liquid in terms of kind, volume, and frequency of intake. Chlorinated water, distilled water, coffee, black tea, herb teas, mineral water and all bubbling waters (carbonated), and hard liquor are preferably avoided, as well as other stimulant and aromatic beverages, and sugared and soft drinks.

Kinds of Beverages

Regular Use

Bancha twig tea (kukicha)
Bancha stem tea
Roasted barley tea
Roasted brown rice tea
Spring water
Well water

Occasional Use

Grain coffee
Dandelion tea
Kombu tea
Umeboshi tea

Burdock root tea
Lotus root tea
Mu tea
Amasake
Carrot juice
Celery juice
Sweet vegetable drink
Other traditionally used and commonly consumed non-stimulating, non-aromatic natural herb teas (made from seeds, leaves, stems, bark, or roots)

Less Frequent Use

Green tea
Barley green juice
Vegetable juice
Fruit juice (apple juice, grape juice, apricot juice, and other temperate climate fruit juices) and cider
Beer (more naturally fermented quality)
Wine (more naturally fermented quality)
Sake (fermented rice wine)
Soy milk (preferably prepared with kombu)
Other juices made from fruits and vegetables that have been traditionally grown and consumed in a temperate climate
Other weak alcohol beverages traditionally and commonly consumed

Modifications

In some instances, such as occasional requirement for nutritional balance or special social events, the Standard Macrobiotic Diet can be further modified temporarily to include some other foods such as salmon, tuna, other red-meat or blue-skinned or fatty fish, organic fertilized fowl's eggs, caviar, and other fish eggs, white-meat poultry, cow's skim milk or goat's milk, traditionally fermented cheese and yogurt, unrefined honey, maple syrup, and beet sugar.

These modifications are to be made according to individual requirements and necessity, though within the Standard Macrobiotic

Diet, these foods would not be regularly and commonly recommended in daily practice to maintain health and well being.

Way of Eating

To establish well-being, Standard Macrobiotic Dietary practice recommends the following:

1. Eat regularly, two to three meals a day. In the case of vigorous physical activity, the frequency of meals may be increased to four times a day.

2. Every meal should include grain or grain products. Grain and grain products ideally comprise about 50 percent of the daily intake of food.

3. Variety in food selection and preparation, proper combinations of foods, and proper cooking are essential.

4. Cooking is to be done with a peaceful mind, with love, and with care.

5. Snacks are to be taken in moderation. They should not replace a regular meal.

6. Beverages may be consumed comfortably as desired.

7. Refrain from eating before bedtime, preferable three hours, to allow for proper digestion.

8. Chew each mouthful very well, at least fifty times, until it becomes liquid.

9. Volume of food varies according to individual need.

10. Eat with the spirit of gratitude and appreciation for all people, society, nature, and the universe as a whole.

Way of Life Suggestions

The following way of life practices will further contribute to our health and happiness:

1. Live each day happily without being preoccupied with your health. Try to keep mentally and physically active.

2. View everything and everyone you meet with gratitude, particularly offering thanks before and after every meal.

3. It is best to get up early every morning and go to bed before midnight.

4. It is best to wear cotton and other natural fiber clothing, especially for undergarments, and to use cotton bed sheets and pillows. Avoid synthetic or woolen clothing directly on the skin and avoid excessive metallic accessories on the fingers, wrists, or neck. Keep such ornaments simple and graceful.

5. If your strength permits, go outdoors in simple clothing. Walk on the grass, beach, or soil up to one half hour each day. Keep your home in good order, from the kitchen, bathroom, bedroom, and living rooms, to every corner.

6. Initiate and maintain an active correspondence, extending your best wishes to parents, children, brothers and sisters, teachers, and friends.

7. Avoid taking long, hot baths or showers unless you have been consuming too much salt or animal food, as these take minerals from the body.

8. If your condition permits, exercise regularly as part of daily life, including activities like walking, scrubbing floors, cleaning windows, washing clothes, and working in the garden. You may also participate in exercise programs such as yoga, martial arts, dance, or sports.

9. Avoid using electric cooking devices (including blenders, ovens, and ranges) or microwave ovens that adversely affect the quality and vibration of the food. Convert to gas or wood stove cooking at the earliest opportunity.

10. It is best to minimize the frequent use of color television and computers.

11. Include some large green plants in your house to freshen and enrich the oxygen content of the air of your home.

12. Sing a happy song every day.

Sample Recipes

The following recipes are examples from the Standard Macrobiotic Diet. Please refer to the cookbooks in the Recommended Reading list for a complete variety of dishes, and please attend cooking classes for instruction in actual preparation of foods.

Brown Rice

1. Soak 2 cups of washed organically grown brown rice in 3 cups of spring water for 3 to 5 hours or overnight.
2. Place in a pressure cooker with a pinch of sea salt or a 1-inch piece of kombu sea vegetable per cup of rice.
3. Bring up to pressure on a medium high flame.
4. When pressure is up, place a flame deflector underneath and lower the flame.
5. Cook for 50 minutes.
6. Turn off the flame and let the pressure reduce itself naturally.
7. Remove the rice from the pot and put in a wooden bowl.

Other combinations of grains

For variety, you can combine 80 percent brown rice with 20 percent barley or 80 percent brown rice with 20 percent millet or wheat berries or corn, etc. Combinations of grains and beans: 90 percent brown rice with 10 percent azuki beans, or 90 percent brown rice with 10 percent black soybeans or chickpeas.

Morning Cereal

A delicious morning porridge can be made by pressure cooking or boiling rice, millet, barley, or other grain using 5 cups of water to 1 cup of grain and by seasoning and cooking as above.

Noodles in Broth

1. Bring 6 to 8 cups of spring water to a boil.
2. Add 1 8-ounce package of udon (whole wheat) or soba (whole wheat and buckwheat) noodles and return to a boil.
3. After about 10 minutes check to see if they are done by breaking the end of one noodle. Soba cooks faster than udon and thinner noodles faster than thicker. If the inside and outside are the same color, the noodles are ready.
4. When done, remove the noodles from the pot, drain, and rinse thoroughly with cold water to prevent clumping.
5. Meanwhile, for the broth, put 1 piece of kombu, 2 to 3 inches long, in a pot and add fresh water.
6. Soak 2 dried shiitake mushrooms, cut off and discard their stems, and slice the mushrooms. Add them to the pot, bring to boil, lower the heat, and simmer for 3 to 5 minutes.
7. Remove the kombu and shiitake and use in other dishes.
8. Add soy sauce (shoyu) to taste to the pot and cook for 3 to 5 minutes.
9. Put the cooked noodles into the broth to warm them, but do not let them boil.
10. When hot, remove the noodles and serve immediately with a little broth. Garnish with scallions, chives, or toasted nori.

Note: If desired, add a little grated fresh ginger to the broth. Also cooked seitan, tofu, tempeh, or natto may be enjoyed with noodles and broth.

Sourdough Bread

1. To make starter, combine 1 cup of wholewheat flour and enough water to make a thick batter.
2. Cover with damp cloth and allow to ferment for 3 to 4 days in a warm place.
3. After starter has soured, add 1 to 1 1/2 cups of starter to bread dough.
4. This dough is made by mixing 8 cups wholewheat flour, 1/4 to 1/2 teaspoon sea salt, and 2 tablespoons sesame oil, and sifting thoroughly together by hand.
5. Form a ball of dough by adding just enough water and knead 300 to 350 times.
6. Oil two bread pans with sesame oil and place dough in pans.

7. Place damp cloth over pans and let sit for 8 to 12 hours in a warm place.

8. After dough has risen, bake at 300 degrees for 15 minutes and then 1 hour and 15 minutes longer at 350 degrees.

Miso Soup

1. Soak wakame sea vegetable (1 1/2-inch piece per person) for 5 minutes and then cut into small pieces.

2. Add to cold water and bring to a boil. Meanwhile, cut vegetables into small pieces.

3. Add the vegetables to the boiling broth and boil all together for 2 to 4 minutes until vegetables are soft and edible.

4. Dilute miso (1/2 to 1 flat teaspoon per cup of broth), add to soup, and simmer for 3 to 4 minutes on a low flame.

5. Occasionally a small portion of shiitake mushrooms can be included with the other vegetables.

Note: Please vary the types of vegetables every day and include leafy greens often.

Other Soup Suggestions

1. Grain and Vegetable Soup: Add leftover cooked grains to basic miso soup or make fresh millet or barley soup with vegetables.

2. Bean and Vegetable Soup: Add leftover cooked beans to basic miso soup or make a fresh soup using lentils, chickpeas, or pre-cooked beans.

3. Squash Soup: Cut and cook butternut, buttercup, acorn, or other fall-season squash in water until it dissolves. Season with a pinch of sea salt or a dash of soy sauce (shoyu).

Other Soup Seasoning Suggestions

1. Light use of soy sauce (shoyu).
2. Light graceful use of sea salt.
Note: Add small amount of fresh garnish when serving (chopped parsley or scallions). Please try and use fresh soup every day and avoid using too many leftovers.

Boiled Vegetables (Nishime style waterless cooking)

1. Use a heavy pot with a heavy lid or cookware specifically designed for waterless cooking.
2. Soak a 3-inch piece of kombu until soft and cut into 1-inch square pieces.
3. Place kombu in bottom of pot and cover with water (about 1 to 2 inches)
4. Add sliced vegetables. For nishime preparation, vegetables are cut in large size. It is usually a combination of 2 or 3 such as carrots or daikon or turnip or burdock root, and onions, hard winter squash or cabbage may also be added.
5. The vegetables can then be layered in the pot, on top of the kombu or placed in sections around the pot.
6. Sprinkle a small volume of sea salt or soy sauce (shoyu) over the vegetables.
7. Cover and set flame on high until a good steam is generated. Lower the flame and cook peacefully for 15 to 20 minutes. If the water should evaporate too quickly during cooking, add more water to the bottom of the pot.
8. When each vegetable has become soft and edible, add a few drops of soy sauce (shoyu) and shake the pot (rather than stirring).
9. Cover again and cook over a low flame for 3 to 5 minutes more.
10. Remove cover, turn off flame and let the vegetables sit for about 2 minutes. You may serve the vegetable juice along with the dish as it is very delicious.

Combination Suggestions:

1. Carrot/burdock and kombu
2. Burdock/lotus root and kombu
3. Daikon/lotus root and kombu
4. Carrot/parsnip and kombu
5. Turnip/shiitake mushroom and kombu
6. Squash/onion and kombu.

Aduki Beans with Squash and Kombu

1. Wash and soak 1/2 cup of azuki beans with a 1-inch square piece of kombu for 2 to 5 hours.

2. Place kombu in bottom of the pot and add chopped hard winter squash such as acorn, butternut, or buttercup. When squash is not available, substitute onions, carrots, or parsnips.

3. Add azuki beans on top of squash and cover with water.

4. Cook over a low flame until the beans and squash become soft. While cooking, you may need to add cold water for a few times.

5. When beans are 80 percent done, add a few pinches of sea salt.

6. Cover and let cook another 10 to 15 minutes or until all the water has cooked down.

7. Turn off the flame and let the pot sit for several minutes before serving.

Note: During cooking, it is best not to stir the beans.

Tofu or Tempeh Stew

1. Soak a 4-inch piece of kombu in 3 cups of spring water.

2. Bring to a boil and cook for 3 to 5 minutes.

3. Add either tofu or tempeh sliced into 1/2-inch cubes along with sliced daikon, carrots, lotus root, or other root vegetables and cook for about 15 minutes.

4. Add two or three of the following: onions, cabbage or Chinese cabbage, squash or Brussel sprouts, and cook for 3 to 5 minutes.

5. If you use fresh tofu, add it with the lighter green vegetables toward the end of cooking.

7. Chop finely 2 or 3 scallions and cook in for 1 minute.

Note: All vegetables should be boiled and cooked until soft, but the greens should still be fresh. A small amount of ginger may be added at the very end of cooking. A mild seasoning of miso may be added at the end instead of soy sauce.

Steamed Greens

1. Wash and slice any of the following: turnip greens, daikon greens, carrot tops, kale, collard greens, mustard greens, watercress, Chinese cabbage.

2. Place the vegetables in a small amount of water (from 1/4 to 1/2 inch) or in a stainless steal steamer over 1 inch of boiling water.

3. Cover and steam for 2 to 3 minutes, depending on the texture of the vegetables.

4. At the end of cooking, lightly sprinkle with soy sauce (shoyu) and serve.

Note: When served, greens should be fresh and bright.

Arame or Hiziki with Carrots and Onions

1. Wash arame or hiziki in cold water, place in bowl for 10 minutes, and put in a strainer to drain.

2. Oil a skillet with 1 tablespoon dark sesame oil.

3. Sauté 1 medium sliced carrot and 1/2 cup onions, sliced in half moons, for 1 to 2 minutes, stirring to ensure even cooking.

4. Add the arame or hiziki on top and enough water to just cover the onions and a tablespoon of soy sauce (shoyu).

5. Cover and bring to a boil, then turn flame to medium-low, and simmer for about 20 minutes.

6. Add more soy sauce to taste.

7. Simmer for 10 to 15 minutes and then mix until the liquid has evaporated.

Sautéed Vegetables

1. Cut carrots, onions, cabbage (finely cut), or other vegetables, including leafy green vegetables.

2. Brush the bottom of the pan with dark sesame oil or put just a small amount of water. When hot, sauté the vegetables quickly for a few minutes. Sprinkle with a pinch of sea salt or soy sauce (shoyu) and add a little water if necessary.

3. Simmer for a few more minutes. The vegetables should be crispy and colorful but cooked.

Boiled Salad

When making a boiled salad, boil each vegetable in the same water but separately. Cook the mildest tasting vegetables first, so that each will retain its distinctive flavor. Any combination of two or three vegetables may be used, making sure it is varied frequently. For this one-minute cooking style, the vegetables are to be chopped in matchsticks or thin slices.

1. Place several inches of water and a pinch of sea salt in a pot and bring to a boil.

2. Drop in a small amount of vegetables at a time and allow to boil for 1 minute. Remove quickly from water and place in a strainer.

3. Repeat as above with each kind of vegetable. When done, place in a serving dish.

Note: The vegetables in this dish are fresh and crispy. They may be served plain or with either a few drops of vinegar (brown rice or umeboshi) or condiments.

Gomashio (Toasted Sesame Seed Salt)

The standard ratio for gomashio is 1 part salt to 16 parts sesame seeds and can be varied depending on individual needs.

1. In a stainless steel skillet, toast the sea salt for a few minutes until it is shiny and then grind it well in a suribachi until very fine.

2. Place washed sesame seeds in the skillet and toast on a low medium flame, stirring constantly with a wooden spoon, shaking the skillet from time to time. When the seeds give off a nutty fragrance and begin popping, crush one between the thumb and fourth finger (it should crush easily).

3. Place the seeds in a Japanese style mortar (suribachi) containing the ground sea salt and slowly grind with an even circular motion until each seed is half crushed.

4. Allow to cool down and store in a covered glass jar.

Quick Soy Sauce Pickles

1. Slice root or round vegetables 1/8-inch thick and cover with a mixture of 1/2 water and 1/2 soy sauce (shoyu).

2. After 2 hours (or less with onions), remove vegetables from the liquid and serve. If taste is too salty, rinse quickly.

3. Reuse the liquid in future pickling.

Cooked Apples

1. Wash several organically grown apples, slice, and place in a pot with a small amount of water to keep from burning (about 1/4 to 1/2 cup).
2. Add pinch of sea salt and simmer for 10 minutes or until soft.

Other Fruit: for variety, try apricots, peaches, blueberries, or other temperate-climate fruit.

Amasake Pudding

1. Place 1 quart amasake and 6 tablespoons kuzu diluted in a little water in a pot.
2. Stir and slowly bring to a boil.
3. Continue to stir constantly to avoid lumping and burning.
4. Simmer for 2 to 3 minutes, remove from heat, and pour into a serving dish.
5. Smooth the amaske and garnish with a slice of lemon and a few fresh green leaves in the center of the dish. Allow to set before serving. If enough kuzu is used to thicken the amasake, it will harden and can be cut into squares.

Variations:

For a different pudding, raisins, apples, apricots, pears, peaches, strawberries, and other sliced fresh fruit may be cooked with the amasake before adding the kuzu. Squash purée or chestnut purée also goes well in this dessert.

Bancha Tea

1. Add about 2 tablespoons of roasted twigs to 1 1/2 quarts of spring water and bring to a boil.
2. Lower flame and simmer for several minutes.
3. Place bamboo tea strainer in cup and pour out tea. Twigs in strainer may be returned to teapot.

Appendix

Dietary Guidelines for Tropical and Semitropical Regions

Traditionally, in South Asia, Southeast Asia, Africa, Central and South America, and other tropical and semitropical regions, people have been eating cooked whole cereal grains as principal food. The grain, including long-grain rice, basmati rice, sorghum, and others, is complemented with vegetables, as well as soup and broth, beans and sea vegetables, and other categories of food in the Standard Macrobiotic Diet.

Proportions of foods, cooking styles, seasoning, and other factors may differ from standard cooking in temperate regions. For example, the amount of vegetables, fresh raw salad, and fruit may be slightly higher; steaming, stir-frying, braising, and other lighter cooking methods may be used more frequently, including boiling of grain rather than pressure-cooking; and less salt, miso, soy sauce or lighter miso and other seasonings may be used. However, in a hot and humid climate, a salty taste may often be more required than in a temperate climate.

In addition to whole grains, some cultures and island societies such as Hawaii and the Caribbean islands have traditionally consumed cassava, taro, yams, sweet potatoes, and other roots and tubers as staple food. In such cases, these may be included in the grain category as the principal source of complex carbohydrates.

In addition to fish and seafood, a small volume of wild animals, birds, and insects may be eaten if traditionally and commonly consumed. Also a small volume of spices, herbs, and aromatic, fragrant

59

beverages may be taken on occasion to help offset the high heat and humidity. Typical foods in tropical and semitropical regions include:

Whole Grains and Staple Roots and Tubers

Long-grain brown rice
Medium-grain brown rice
Basmati rice
Sorghum
Barley
Corn
Amaranth
Quinoa
Teff
Bulghur
Couscous
Sweet potato
Yam
Taro (albi, poi)
Cassava (yuca, manioc, tapioca)
Other grains, grain products, staple roots and tubers that have traditionally been consumed in tropical and semitropical regions

Vegetables from Land and Sea

Artichoke
Asparagus
Avocado
Bamboo shoots
Curly dock
Eggplant
Fennel
Green pepper

Jicama
Okra
Plantain
Purslane
Potato (traditionally processed)
Spinach
Swiss chard
Zucchini

Other vegetables that have traditionally been consumed in tropical and semitropical regions

Sea Vegetables, Water Moss, River and Lake Moss

Fruit, Nuts, and Seeds

Banana	Mango
Breadfruit	Orange
Coconut	Papaya
Grapefruit	Pineapple
Guava	Plantain
Kiwi	Quince
All seeds and nuts	Tangerine

Other fruits that have traditionally been consumed in tropical and semitropical regions

Dietary Guidelines for Polar and Semipolar Regions

Traditionally, in Alaska, Northern Canada, Greenland, Iceland, Scandinavia, Northern Russia, Siberia, Mongolia, Tibet, the Andes, and other cold climates and regions, the standard diet has included proportionately more animal food than in temperate latitudes. Because of the short growing season, grains and vegetables are in shorter supply, though traditionally hardy strains of buckwheat, mountain barley, and other grains were harvested, as well as a wide variety of wild plants (including wild burdock, milkweed, dandelion, mugwort, wild leek, water lily root, wild ginger, and wild beans), sea vegetables and mosses, fruits (including chokeberry, wild cherry, currants, cranberries, blueberries, wild strawberries, and grapes), seeds and nuts (such as acorns), and roots, stems, leaves, and flowers of many kinds.

In addition to slightly more fish and seafood (on average from 20 to 30 percent of the daily diet, especially in colder seasons), people in polar and semipolar regions ate a small amount of whale, caribou, wild game, and dairy food. Because of the cold weather and hard physical activity, they were able to digest small amounts of these foods without ill effects as is the case in other climates and environments and among people observing a more sedentary lifestyle. Further, pressure-cooking, long-time boiling, broiling, baking, roasting, and other stronger cooking methods may be used more frequently; and more salt, miso, soy sauce (shoyu), and other seasonings as well as darker miso may be used.

Recommended Reading

The Book of Macrobiotics by Michio Kushi, Japan Publications, revised edition, 1987. *The best general introduction to macrobiotic philosophy and way of life. Includes complete nutritional tables on macrobiotic quality foods.*

Macrobiotic Diet by Michio and Aveline Kushi, Japan Publications, 1985. *An indepth look at the standard diet, including nutritional balance, food history, explanation of cooking methods, and special dishes.*

Aveline Kushi's Complete Guide to Macrobiotic Cooking by Aveline Kushi, Warner Books, 1985. *Aveline's basic cookbook for health and happiness enlived by stories, poems, and drawings about her early life in Japan.*

Aveline Kushi's Introducing Macrobiotic Cooking by Wendy Esko, Japan Publications, revised edition, 1987. *A popular introduction to macrobiotic cooking.*

Changing Seasons Cookbook by Aveline Kushi and Wendy Esko, Avery Publishing Group, 1985. *How to cook according to seasonal change.*

The Cancer-Prevention Diet by Michio Kushi and Alex Jack, St. Martin's Press, 1983. *The major book on the macrobiotic approach to degenerative disease, including dietary recommendations for the twenty-five most common cancers.*

Diet for a Strong Heart by Michio Kushi and Alex Jack, St. Martin's Press, 1985. *The macrobiotic approach to heart attack, stroke, high blood pressure, and other cardiovascular disease.*

Doctors Look at Macrobiotics, edited by Edward Esko, Japan Publications, 1988. *Ten medical doctors describe the benefits of macrobiotics in their personal and professional life.*

Let Food Be Thy Medicine by Alex Jack, One Peaceful World Press, 1991. *Digest of 185 scientific and medical studies showing the benefits of the macrobiotic dietary approach on personal health, family health, and the environment.*

Macrobiotic Home Remedies by Michio Kushi and Marc Van Cauwenberghe, M.D., Japan Publications, 1985. *Guide to traditional home cares and external applications.*

Food Governs Your Destiny: The Teachings of Namboku Mizuno, translated by Michio and Aveline Kushi, Japan Publications, 1991. *The pithy teachings of an 18th century Japanese physiognomist and philosopher.*

Macrobiotic Family Favorites by Aveline Kushi and Wendy Esko, Japan Publications, 1988. *Tasty menus and recipes for children and teenagers.*

Macrobiotic Child Care and Family Health by Michio and Aveline Kushi, Japan Publications, 1986. *How to raise healthy children and create family unity.*

One Peaceful World by Michio Kushi and Alex Jack, St. Martin's Press, 1987. *Michio Kushi's autobiography and guide to a peaceful mind, home, and world community.*

Nine Star Ki by Michio Kushi and Edward Esko. *An introduction to Oriental astrology and cosmology and guidebook on love and relationships, health and travel, and getting through the 1990s.*

These and other macrobiotic books are available at natural foods stores and book stores. They are also available by mail order directly from One Peaceful World Press. Please use or copy the form on the following page and send it with your order.

Mail Order Form for Books

Title	Price	Quantity
Standard Macrobiotic Diet	$5.95	_____
The Book of Macrobiotics	$15.95	_____
Macrobiotic Diet	$15.95	_____
Aveline Kushi's Complete Guide	$13.95	_____
Aveline Kushi's Introducing	$14.95	_____
Changing Seasons Cookbook	$12.95	_____
The Cancer-Prevention Diet	$10.95	_____
Diet for a Strong Heart	$10.95	_____
Doctors Look at Macrobiotics	$14.95	_____
Let Food Be Thy Medicine	$10.95	_____
Macrobiotic Home Remedies	$14.95	_____
Food Governs Your Destiny	$12.95	_____
Macrobiotic Family Favorites	$15.95	_____
Macrobiotic Child Care	$15.95	_____
One Peaceful World	$12.95	_____
Nine Star Ki	$12.95	_____

Subtotal _____

Postage ($1.50 first book and .50 each additional book) _____

TOTAL _____

___Enclosed is my check/money order payable to OPW Press

___Bill my ___Visa ___MasterCard #_____Exp. Date_____

Signature_____

Ship to:

_____

_____

_____

For information on bulk purchases at special discount, please write to OPW. Prices subject to change. Foreign orders, please pay in U.S. funds and add 20% of total for surface postage and 35% for airmail.

One Peaceful World Press
Box 10
Becket, MA 01223 U.S.A.